RESUSCITATION OF BABIES AT BIRTH

RESUSCITATION OF BABIES AT BIRTH

A Report of a Joint Working Party of the Royal College of Paediatrics and Child Health and The Royal College of Obstetricians and Gynaecologists.

This handbook has been produced by nominated representatives of:

The Royal College of Paediatrics and Child Health (formerly the British Paediatric Association)
The British Association of Perinatal Medicine
The Royal College of Anaesthetists
The Royal College of Midwives
The Royal College of Obstetricians and Gynaecologists
The Neonatal Nurses Association
and has been endorsed by their Councils.
It has also been endorsed by the European Resuscitation Council.

This handbook is intended to replace the previous handbook on resuscitation of the newborn produced by a similar working party (1989), and takes account of developments in practice and teaching.

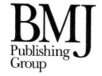

BMJ
Publishing
Group

First published in 1997
by the BMJ Publishing Group, BMA House, Tavistock Square,
London WC1H 9JR

British Library Cataloguing in Publication Data

A catalogue record for this book is available from the British Library

ISBN 0–7279–1179–1

Typeset by Apek Typesetters, Nailsea, Bristol
Printed and bound by Latimer Trend, Plymouth

Contents

Working party members

Dr Patricia Hamilton (Chair), Consultant in Neonatal Paediatrics, St George's Hospital Medical School, London *(Royal College of Paediatrics and Child Health)*

Mrs Lesley Doherty, Conference Chairperson *(Neonatal Nurses Association)*

Ms Catherine McCormick, Midwifery Liaison Manager *(Royal College of Midwives)*

Professor James Neilson, Professor of Obstetrics and Gynaecology, University of Liverpool *(Royal College of Obstetricians and Gynaecologists)*

Dr Sam Richmond, Consultant Paediatrician, Sunderland General Hospital *(Royal College of Paediatrics and Child Health)*

Dr Andrew Wilkinson, Reader in Paediatrics and Perinatal Medicine, University of Oxford John Radcliffe Hospital, Oxford *(British Association of Perinatal Medicine)*

Dr David Zideman, Consultant Anaesthetist, Hammersmith Hospital, London *(Royal College of Anaesthetists, European Resuscitation Council)*

Acknowledgements

Many people have made helpful comments during the progress of this document.

The working group would particularly like to thank the Northern Neonatal Network for use of material from their booklet and St George's Hospital Medical School Audio-visual Unit for preparation of the figures.

Time is of the utmost importance. *Delay* is damaging to the infant. *Act* promptly, accurately and gently.

Virginia Apgar

1 Introduction

We recognise that there are many controversies in neonatal resuscitation and there is not always evidence available to resolve them, so there is clearly a need for further research. This handbook amounts to a collection of widely (but not necessarily universally) accepted opinion. What follows is a guide to resuscitation at birth. It should not be regarded as a rigid protocol, but as a way of proceeding that is thought to be both safe and effective by many in the field, based on experience, current evidence and research.

This handbook is not a textbook of physiology although, where possible, some theoretical basis is given and suggestions for further reading made for those who wish to review the evidence. It is not anticipated that the text will be consulted during resuscitation itself. The accompanying resuscitation charts (1 and 2) are designed for guidance at the place of birth (see pp 57, 58).

We hope that this text will be thoroughly read and that the guidelines will form the template for locally agreed policies to be followed by any professional who may be involved in resuscitation of babies at birth.

The British Paediatric Association (BPA) working party report, 'Neonatal Resuscitation' (June 1993)[1], outlined many of the principles of neonatal resuscitation and made recommendations for training in resuscitation and the personnel who should be available where babies are delivered.

Successful resuscitation requires the coordinated efforts of midwives, doctors and nurses. The precise role of professionals within the team will vary according to local circumstances. All midwives and junior doctors should be competent in lung inflation and ventilation via a mask. Tracheal intubation should only be undertaken by those trained in its use and with sufficient practice to maintain the skill. However, all team members must understand the procedure and be able to assist.

Local training arrangements must ensure that individuals are competent to fulfil their team roles and involve practice in working together as well as in specific skills.

2 General principles

The majority of newborn babies will establish normal breathing and circulation spontaneously. They will need only attention to the maintenance of their temperature and perhaps gentle stimulation to start breathing. Some may need suctioning of the airway and a few will need assisted lung inflation via a mask. Fewer still may need tracheal intubation. Very few indeed will need external chest compression and intervention with drugs.

Nevertheless, it is essential that trained and experienced healthcare personnel are available for every delivery.

2.1 Normal physiology

It is recommended that the reader is familiar with the physiological mechanisms of the first breath, reabsorption of lung fluid and establishment of a functional residual volume. In addition, it is helpful to have a good understanding of the changes that occur during the transition from fetal circulation (see Recommended reading).

2.1.1 The first breath

The lungs actively secrete fluid in utero and at term contain approximately 30 ml of fluid per kilogram body weight.

The first few breaths must overcome the surface tension present within the lung, drive any residual fluid from the alveoli into the circulation and fill the lungs with air. Once the initial opening pressure has been achieved, subsequent breaths do not need to be so forceful. Provided that sufficient surfactant is present, the baby rapidly establishes a residual volume so the lungs do not collapse completely at the end of exhalation and less effort is required for subsequent inflations. The ability of the fetus to produce pulmonary surfactant increases with increasing gestational age. Surfactant production is rapidly reduced by cold stress and by acidosis.

2.1.2 Circulatory changes

In utero, little blood flows to the lungs because of high resistance in the pulmonary circulation and lower resistance to flow into the aorta and placenta. Most of the blood leaving the right ventricle passes from the pulmonary artery into the aorta via the ductus arteriosus. Resistance to flow into the aorta increases after the umbilical vessels are clamped and resistance to flow into the pulmonary circulation rapidly falls following lung expansion. As a result, blood leaving the right ventricle passes into the pulmonary circulation and returns via the pulmonary veins into the left atrium. These changes result in closure of the foramen ovale and the ductus arteriosus soon after birth.

2.2 Abnormal situations

Any professional attending a delivery must be able to recognise a baby who is not establishing normal respiration and circulation. This will be based on observation of respiratory effort, heart rate, colour and tone (Sections 6.1–6.3). Appropriate resuscitation steps are outlined in this document and are based on the general understanding of what happens in asphyxia as summarised below. It must be emphasised, however, that not all babies born in poor condition at birth have been subjected to perinatal asphyxia, and asphyxia should not be assumed to be the cause without good reason to do so.

2.2.1 Asphyxia

Animal studies have shown that a severe abrupt lack of oxygen at birth initially causes arrest of breathing movements – primary apnoea. There is a rapid rise in blood pressure accompanied by slowing of the heart rate, and hence reduced cardiac output, with a rise in peripheral vascular resistance accompanied by secretion of catecholamines, vasopressin, angiotensin and other hormones. Blood flow to essential fetal organs (heart and brain) is maintained at the expense of all other organs including the lungs, where vasoconstriction occurs. This period of primary apnoea continues for a variable time. Deep agonal gasping then begins and occurs about every 10–20 seconds.

If hypoxia continues, gasping fades away and there is a second apnoeic phase – terminal apnoea. At the same time, blood

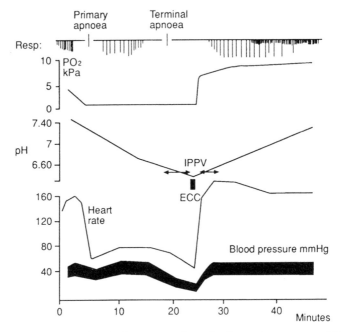

Figure 2.1. Physiological stages of asphyxia and recovery. (After Northern Neonatal Network. *Principles of Resuscitation at Birth*, 1996). ECC = external chest compression; IPPV = intermittent positive pressure ventilation.

pressure begins to fall, heart rate decreases still further and, without intervention, death ensues (Figure 2.1).

A baby who does not breathe within a minute or two of birth may either be in primary apnoea and about to start gasping, or has already progressed through the gasping phase into terminal apnoea before birth. In either case appropriate resuscitation should not be delayed.

In primary apnoea the baby will probably recover with minimal help and will tend to be blue rather than pale, although this is not always a reliable indicator. The heart rate will improve when the airway is clear and air or oxygen enters the lungs. A gasp or two will be taken before the skin becomes pink.

Prolongation of the primary apnoeic phase may be produced by drugs administered to the mother, such as opiates, anaesthetic agents and sedatives.

A baby in terminal apnoea will usually be very pale rather than blue, very floppy and will die unless actively resuscitated. Assisted ventilation is mandatory and the baby will usually become pink before taking a spontaneous gasp.

A strategy for resuscitation can be based on an understanding of these physiological processes.

3 Anticipation

At every delivery there should be at least one person present who is responsible for giving basic care to the baby, initiating resuscitation if necessary and summoning more help if needed. There should always be someone available who has the necessary expertise and who can be summoned immediately for the prompt resuscitation of the baby who unexpectedly needs intervention. In some situations more than one trained person will be needed and close teamwork is essential. Responsibilities should be clearly assigned so that individual roles are understood.

Guidelines are suggested in Appendix A, but local circumstances will dictate the situations when an appropriately trained person should be called to stand by at a delivery in order to resuscitate the baby if necessary. Locally agreed guidelines should take into account the geography and availability of trained personnel, drawn from a team of doctors, midwives or neonatal nurses. The means by which experienced help is summoned must be clearly set out.

Local audit should evaluate these guidelines. There should not be an excessive number of unexpected emergency calls and nor should time be wasted in too many unnecessary attendances. Any untoward events should be reviewed.

4 Equipment

A list of items of equipment that should be available is given in Appendix B, and the appropriate equipment checks in Appendix C. Responsibility for these equipment checks should be agreed locally.

5 Preparation before the baby is born

Keep the delivery room warm (as close to 25°C as possible) and the doors closed to reduce draughts.

Check the mother's case records (and the baby's if available) and make yourself known to the parents if you have not previously met them.

Consider whether you need an assistant or the support of a more experienced colleague, particularly for extremely preterm babies, multiple deliveries or those where severe problems are anticipated.

Wash your hands and put on gloves.

Check all the equipment (Appendix C).

Even a vigorous newborn baby may experience a marked fall in body temperature when exposed. A compromised baby or a preterm baby is at particular risk from cold stress. To reduce heat loss:

Keep the delivery room warm.

Ensure prewarmed towels are available.

Switch on the radiant heater in case resuscitation is needed.

6 Procedure after the baby is born

Start the **clock**.

Receive the baby, remove the wet towels and dry with a warm towel.

Cover the baby with a warm towel to minimise heat loss.

Assess:

1. Breathing. Observe the rate and quality of the respirations, and particularly note any abnormal breathing pattern such as grunting or gasping.

2. Heart rate. Assess the rate and quality of the pulse by listening to the apex beat with a stethoscope and palpating the pulse at the base of the umbilical cord.

3. Colour. Note if the baby is centrally pink, cyanosed or pale. Look at the trunk, lips and tongue. Peripheral cyanosis is common and does **not** by itself indicate hypoxaemia.

Most healthy mature babies will breathe or cry within 90 seconds of birth and have good muscle tone. Suction of the pharynx is **not** usually necessary and additional oxygen is not required.

Do not leave the baby unnecessarily exposed.

A baby can usually be assigned to one of the three categories described below:

6.1 Breathing spontaneously *and* has a heart rate of > 100 beats/minute *and* is centrally pink

Give to the mother.

If possible the mother should receive the baby straight away. The baby will usually stay warm with skin-to-skin contact and may be put to the breast at this stage.

6.2 Breathing inadequately *but* has a heart rate > 100 beats/minute and is centrally cyanosed

Wrap in a warm dry towel, place under the radiant heater.

Drying the baby usually produces enough stimulation to induce effective breathing but additional safe methods of stimulation include flicking the soles of the feet or gently rubbing the infant's skin. Offer supplementary oxygen. If there is no response, begin more active intervention as set out below.

6.3 Breathing inadequately after stimulation *or* has a heart rate < 100 beats/minute *or* is pale

This baby will need further resuscitation promptly. The steps outlined in the sections below should be followed.

It is highly desirable to have at least two trained practitioners present when there is no response to basic measures.

Call for assistance early if you think you may need it.

The following sections follow the three basic steps in resuscitation:

Airway
Breathing
Circulation

7 Airway

Position the baby face upwards on the resuscitation surface, head towards you. A head-down slope is not necessary. The head should be supported in a neutral position and the jaw drawn forward in order to keep the tongue from obstructing the back of the pharynx. A folded towel placed under the neck and shoulders may help to maintain the neutral position. Beware of over-extension of the neck which can obstruct the airway and is a common cause of problems (Figure 7.1).

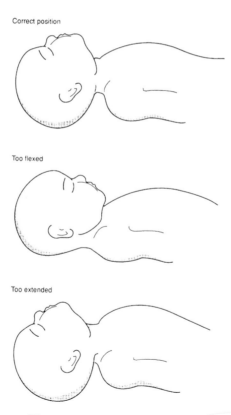

Correct position

Too flexed

Too extended

Figure 7.1. Positioning the airway.

7.1 If there is no meconium in the amniotic fluid

Watch for respiratory efforts and listen to the chest.

If efforts are present and vigorous but no breath sounds are audible the airway may be **obstructed**. **Check** the position of the baby and **reposition** if necessary.

Gently **suction** the mouth and nostrils to remove debris or mucus. Use a 10FG (or, if preterm, an 8FG) suction catheter connected to a suction source with a negative pressure not exceeding −100 mmHg (13.3 kPa). The catheter should not be inserted too far into the oropharynx and should not touch the back wall of the pharynx, as this may result in bradycardia and apnoea. Each attempt at suction should continue for no longer than 5 seconds. Manual suction devices with a trap, or preferably a mechanical device, should be used to prevent contamination of the operator. The Royal College of Obstetricians and Gynaecologists' guidelines on protection against HIV infection should be followed[2].

Excessive, persistent secretions may occur with oesophageal atresia, a condition where the outcome may be improved by early detection. The diagnosis may be confirmed by attempting to pass a wide-bore nasogastric tube.

7.2 If the airway still appears to be obstructed

Congenital abnormalities such as choanal atresia (very rare) or Pierre Robin sequence (micrognathia, glossoptosis and cleft palate) should be considered. Both these situations may be helped by the insertion of an oral airway, and babies with Pierre Robin sequence may improve if turned prone. Check for improvement and, if necessary, proceed to tracheal intubation (Section 10.2).

7.3 If there is thick meconium in the airway (Section 15.1.2)

Suction the mouth before delivery of the chest. Suction the mouth and then the nose, trying to avoid inducing a gasp, and proceed as in Section 15.1.2.

8 Breathing

8.1 If respiratory efforts are shallow or slow

Count the heart rate over 10–15 seconds (Section 9.1).

If there is a regular heart rate of > 100 beats/minute and no meconium is present

Stimulate gently and offer supplementary oxygen, through a mask and Y-piece, if the baby is cyanosed. Usually the baby will start to breathe spontaneously.

*If respirations do not improve within a further 20–30 seconds and the heart rate is **decreasing** or the baby remains **cyanosed***

Start lung inflation using a Y-piece and mask or bag, valve and mask (Section 10.1). Ensure that the chest wall moves with each attempt at inflation. Naloxone (Section 12.1.5) may be considered at this stage if the mother has recently received an opiate analgesic but **only if the baby has become pink with a good heart rate and is still not breathing**. Naloxone must **not be a substitute** for the application of definitive resuscitative measures.

By this time the baby will be about 2 minutes old and if the heart rate continues to decrease over the next 30 seconds, in spite of adequate mask ventilation, proceed to tracheal intubation (Section 10.2), calling for assistance if necessary.

8.2 If respirations are absent or gasping, persistently shallow or irregular or the heart rate is < 100 beats/minute

Start lung inflation using a Y-piece and mask or bag, valve and mask (Section 10.1). Prepare to perform tracheal intubation (Section 10.2). Call for assistance if necessary.

9 Circulation

9.1 Heart rate

This is an important indicator of the need for, and response to, resuscitation.

Evaluate the heart rate by:

- Auscultation or palpation over the apex of the heart.
- Palpation of the base of the umbilical cord (to check for output).

If the heart rate is:

- > 100 beats/minute – continue assessment.
- < 100 beats/minute and decreasing – start or continue positive pressure ventilation (Section 10). Check technique.
- < 60 beats/minute – start or continue positive pressure ventilation. Check technique. Start external chest compression (Section 11). Consider drugs and volume expansion (Section 12).

The commonest reason for failure of the heart rate to improve is ineffective lung inflation. This should always be checked before resorting to external chest compression.

9.2 Colour

Oxygen should be given if the baby is centrally cyanosed.

Cyanosis may persist even when the baby has an adequate heart rate and respiratory effort. This may be due to persistent pulmonary hypertension or to the presence of a congenital cardiac abnormality. Oxygen should be given until the cause of the cyanosis is determined.

Pallor may be a sign of asphyxia, hypovolaemia or anaemia. If profound pallor does not improve with ventilation give blood, plasma or albumin as appropriate (Section 12.1.3).

10 Positive pressure ventilation

This may be achieved through a mask or by a tracheal tube. Both techniques require skill and practice. Opportunities for regular training must be provided so that these interventions are performed by personnel with both training and experience.

10.1 Lung inflation through a face mask

10.1.1 Procedure

Check that the airway is not obstructed. Reposition the head and suction the mouth and upper airway if necessary. The commonest reasons for failure are over-extending the baby's neck and not lifting the jaw.

Set the pressure relief valve at 30 cmH$_2$O initially.

Apply the right size face mask (Appendix B.5.2). The mask should cover the baby's mouth and nose and be well fitting, so that when tightly applied it does not press on the eyes nor overhang the chin (Figure 10.1). Hold the chin gently forward using a finger on the tip of the mandible, taking care not to press upwards on the soft tissues in the floor of the mouth (Figure 10.2).

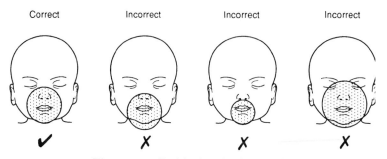

Figure 10.1. Positioning the face mask.

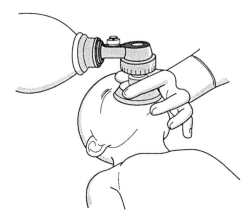

Figure 10.2. Holding the face mask.

10.1.2 If using a Y-piece

Ensure that there is a suitable pressure relief valve and manometer in the circuit. The airway of the baby must never be subjected to an unlimited pressure source because this will result in severe and possibly fatal lung damage.

Occlude the Y-piece (Figure 10.3) for about 2 seconds for the first five or six inflations. After this the chest wall should begin to move with each inflation. Reduce the pressure to about 20 cmH$_2$O

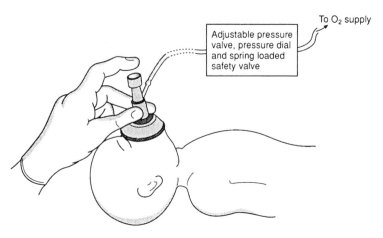

To O$_2$ supply

Adjustable pressure valve, pressure dial and spring loaded safety valve

Figure 10.3. Using a Y-piece, valve and mask.

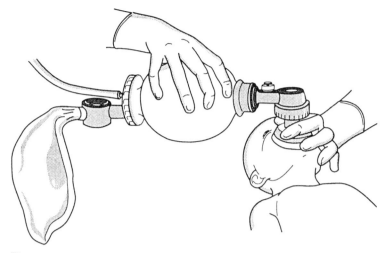

Figure 10.4. Using a bag, valve and mask. Reproduced with permission. *Textbook of Neonatal Resuscitation*. The American Heart Association, 1994

and ventilate the lungs at a rate of 30–40 breaths/minute as above.

10.1.3 If using a resuscitation bag, valve and mask

Squeeze the bag *slowly* with the finger tips (Figure 10.4), trying to maintain inflation times of 1–2 seconds for the first five or six breaths, which should be possible if a 500-ml bag is used. Initial lung inflation may require pressures of 30–40 cmH$_2$O, but once the chest wall is moving pressures of 20 cmH$_2$O should be sufficient. The chest wall should be seen to move by the fifth inflation. After five inflation breaths, check that the chest wall is moving and then ventilate the lungs at a rate of **30–40 breaths/ minute.**

Watch for symmetrical chest wall motion and **listen** for breath and heart sounds.

If the chest wall fails to rise and fall synchronously with inflations:

- **Check** that the mask is applied properly to the face.
- **Check** that the airway is not obstructed. Reposition and suction if necessary, ensuring that the jaw is adequately held forward.
- If still failing to ventilate, **increase** the inflation pressure in steps up to 40 cmH$_2$O.

If the heart rate is > 100 beats/minute and increasing, continue ventilation until spontaneous respiration is established

Once chest expansion has occurred and the heart rate is satisfactory, ventilatory inspiratory pressure should be **reduced** to 15–20 cmH$_2$O, provided that this results in adequate chest wall movement.

If the heart rate is > 100 beats/minute and not increasing, proceed to tracheal intubation (Section 10.2)

If the heart rate decreases to < 60 beats/minute, start **external chest compression** (Section 11) and call for assistance. Prepare to give drugs and volume expanders (Section 12) if the heart rate fails to increase.

10.2 Tracheal intubation

Help will be needed from an assistant to pass appropriate equipment, monitor the baby's condition, attach the ventilation device and summon more assistance if needed.

10.2.1 Procedure

- **Position** the baby with the head in a neutral position (Section 7).
- Gently **insert** the laryngoscope, held in the left hand (Figure 10.5), into the baby's mouth. Guide the blade over the surface

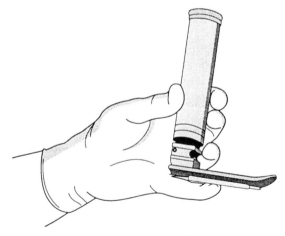

Figure 10.5. Holding the laryngoscope.

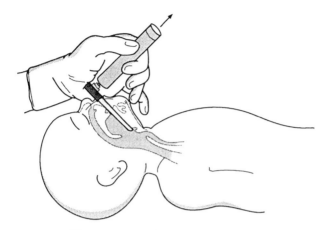

Figure 10.6. Using the laryngoscope.

of the tongue until first the uvula and then the leaf-like epiglottis comes into view. If the blade is inserted too far, only the oesophagus will be seen. If the blade is not inserted far enough then little is seen except the epiglottis. Advance the tip of the blade either into the groove slightly anterior to the epiglottis (the vallecula) or over the epiglottis itself. Lifting the laryngoscope upwards and forwards in the direction of the handle will now bring the larynx into view (Figure 10.6). Gentle upward traction on the laryngoscope handle is required rather than rotation towards the operator. The vocal cords can easily be recognised. Slight external downward pressure on the cricoid cartilage with the fifth finger of the left hand, or by an assistant, will help to bring the larynx into view.

- **Hold** the tracheal tube with the right hand like a pen and gently direct it towards the larynx from the right side of the mouth, keeping the vocal cords in view all the time. Keep the curve of the tube in the horizontal plane so that the view of the larynx is not obscured.

- **Insert** the tip of the tube between the vocal cords and advance it 1–2 cm. The shoulder (Coles type tube) or intubation mark (straight tube) should be positioned just above the cords. As a guide, the distance from the lip to the tip of the tracheal tube should usually be 7, 8 or 9 cm in 1-, 2- or 3-kg babies respectively. Do not force the shoulder of a Coles tube into or through the cords. If the cords are tightly adducted wait for them to relax or for a gasp to occur.

- **Remove** the laryngoscope carefully, holding the tube firmly against the hard palate until it can be carefully secured. Note the length of the tube at the lips and fix it in place. The assistant should now **attach** the tracheal tube either to a Y system or to a resuscitation bag system.
- Give five inflation breaths using about 2 seconds inflation time, then, once the chest wall is moving, ventilate the baby at a rate of 30–40 breaths/minute.
- **Watch** for bilateral and equal chest wall movement and improvement in skin colour.
- **Listen** on both sides of the chest for breath sounds. Listen also for an increase in heart rate.
- **Continue** ventilation until the baby is breathing spontaneously, has a good heart rate and is pink. The tracheal tube may then be removed, but additional oxygen may still be required. If the baby is very preterm or there is any reason for concern, it is advisable to transfer the baby to a neonatal unit for observation before extubation.
- Before intubated transfer, the tube may need to be more firmly secured. It should be fixed in position according to local practice, being careful not to alter the position of the tube whilst doing so.
- **Do not leave** the tracheal tube in place without applying at least 2–3 cm positive end-expiratory pressure to replace the natural expiratory resistance of the larynx.

10.2.2 Possible problems

Intubation attempts should not take more than 30 seconds

If not successful within this time ventilate through a mask before trying again.

If the heart rate is <60 beats/minute

External chest compression (Section 11) should precede and accompany intubation. Prepare to give drugs and consider volume expansion (Section 12) after establishment of ventilation.

If the baby remains cyanosed and the heart rate continues to decrease, consider the following causes

Disconnection of ventilation system
Signs: absent breath sounds, no chest wall movement with inflation.

Action: reconnect system.

Oesophageal intubation
Signs: poor breath sounds, poor chest wall movement, abdominal distension.

Action: **if in any doubt**, reventilate through a mask and then reintubate; ensure the vocal cords are clearly seen before placing the tracheal tube.

Tracheal tube in a main bronchus (usually the right)
Signs: asymmetry of breath sounds and chest wall movement.

Action: slowly withdraw the tube 0·5–1 cm at a time whilst listening in each axilla in turn for equality of breath sounds.

Insufficient inflation pressure
Signs: breath sounds present and symmetrical but poor chest wall movement.

Action: check gas flow and if confident of tube position, increase inflation time and inflation pressure.

Pneumothorax, pleural effusion, diaphragmatic hernia
Signs: persisting asymmetry or absence of breath sounds, chest transillumination (pneumothorax), tense abdomen (pneumothorax), hydrops (pleural effusion), scaphoid abdomen and displaced cardiac apex beat (diaphragmatic hernia).

Action: see Sections 15.2 (pneumothorax), 15.4 (hydrops fetalis), 15.5 (diaphragmatic hernia) – all are very rare.

The baby with bradycardia and cyanosis not responding to intubation and ventilation is in serious trouble – call for assistance sooner rather than later.

11 External chest compression

Start external chest compression if the baby has a heart rate of < 60 beats/minute which is decreasing despite adequate ventilation. The prime purpose of chest compression in neonatal resuscitation is to deliver oxygenated blood to the coronary arteries. This has a beneficial effect on cardiac performance and, if successful, there should be a prompt improvement in heart rate.

Teamwork is essential here, as one person can then attend to ventilating the baby.

The procedure is as follows:

- **Place the thumbs,** side by side or overlapping, over the lower third of the sternum (i.e. just below an imaginary line joining the nipples) with the hands around the chest so that the fingers support the baby's back (Figure 11.1). Alternatively, apply pressure to the same point along the sternum with two fingers whilst the baby is lying supine (Figure 11.2). This latter approach may be more convenient but is known to be less effective[3,4]. The sternum should be compressed by about 2–3 cm in a term baby. The rate should be about 120/minute (2/second) with equal compression and relaxation times.

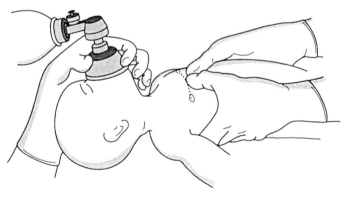

Figure 11.1. External chest compression (preferred method).

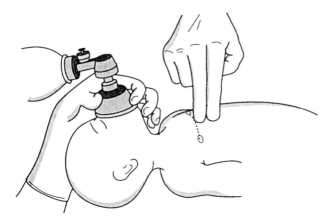

Figure 11.2. External chest compression (alternative method).

- The lungs must be **reinflated** with oxygen after every few compressions. The exact ratio of inflations to cardiac compressions is not critical, provided that it is agreed between those who are doing it. Commonly suggested compressions to inflation ratios include 3:1 and 5:1.
- **Continue** chest compressions until the spontaneous heart rate reaches 80 beats/minute and is increasing.
- **Check** the spontaneous heart rate after 30 seconds. If no response despite good inflation of the lungs and effective chest compression, prepare to give drugs and volume expanders (Section 12). Remember, however, that the commonest cause of a decreasing heart rate is ineffective lung inflation.

12 Medications and fluids

If there is no response to ventilation and external chest compression after 60 seconds, then drugs should be used to try to improve cardiac performance.

12.1 Medications

By this stage of the resuscitation additional assistance should be present. The label of the ampoule and the dose of drug to be given should be checked. A record of drug administration must be kept by a designated member of the team.

12.1.1 Adrenaline

Indications

Heart rate < 60 beats/minute despite external chest compression, tracheal intubation, and effective lung inflation.

Preparation

$1/10\ 000$ dilution ($100\ \mu g/ml$) – for intravenous use.

Dose

$10\ \mu g/kg$ ($0 \cdot 1\ ml/kg$).

Route

Umbilical venous catheter, trachea.

Provided the lungs have been inflated, the first dose may be given via the tracheal tube (Section 12.2.2) whilst preparations are made for umbilical venous catheterisation (Section 12.2.1). It should be remembered that there is little evidence that the tracheal route is effective. The second dose, if needed, should be given via the umbilical venous catheter. A third, larger dose of $100\ \mu g/kg$ may be given intravenously after sodium bicarbonate if still necessary, and after flushing the line carefully again.

12.1.2 Sodium bicarbonate

Indications

Heart rate < 60 beats/minute despite good ventilation, external chest compression and intravenous adrenaline.

Preparation

4·2% solution (0·5 mmol/ml) or 8·4% (1 mmol/ml) diluted with an equal volume of 5–10% dextrose.

Dose

1–2 mmol/kg (2–4 ml/kg of 4·2% solution).

Route

Umbilical venous catheter.

The intention is to deliver base to the coronary arteries to raise myocardial pH, **not** to fully correct the metabolic component of the acidosis. A second dose may be given.

Flush the catheter with 0·9% sodium chloride after administration and particularly before administering any other medication.

12.1.3 Volume expanders

Indications

Hypovolaemia should be considered in any infant who fails to respond to resuscitation, particularly when there is:

- Evidence of acute bleeding.
- Poor response to adequate resuscitation.
- Poor pulse volume.
- Pallor which persists after oxygenation.
- Suspicion of acute severe haemolysis.

Preparations

4–5% human albumin in normal saline (HAS).
Plasma.
Uncross-matched Group O Rhesus negative blood.

Dose

10–20 ml/kg administered over 5–10 minutes, repeated if circulation is poor despite good heart rate.

Route

Umbilical venous catheter, peripheral venous cannula.

12.1.4 Dextrose

Indications

It is not necessary to infuse high concentrations of dextrose – 10% is sufficient to provide a bolus of glucose to the heart.

Preparation

10% dextrose.

Dose

2–3 ml/kg.

Route

Umbilical venous catheter, peripheral venous cannula.

12.1.5 Naloxone hydrochloride

This is an opioid antagonist without respiratory depressant activity. It can reverse apnoea in the baby due to opiates given to the mother in labour.

This is not a drug which improves cardiac performance and should not be given to an asphyxiated baby or any baby whose heart rate is <100 beats/minute.

Indications

Persistent apnoea in an otherwise well baby related to maternal opiate analgesia before delivery.

Naloxone should be reserved for the apnoeic baby whose mother has had repeated doses of opiate analgesia less than 3 hours apart (the adult half life), or who has received opiate analgesia 2–4 hours before delivery. Standard resuscitation should be established first and may be sufficient alone. Naloxone may be given when the airway is secure, ventilation has been achieved and the baby is pink with a good spontaneous heart rate.

Preparations

Naloxone hydrochloride (Narcan) 400 μg/ml.

Dose

100 μg/kg (0.25 ml/kg).

Route

Intramuscular.

Warning

DO NOT give naloxone to the baby of an opiate-dependent mother as this may precipitate severe withdrawal.

12.1.6 Calcium gluconate

There is **no evidence** that calcium is useful in the resuscitation of newborn babies. It is a potent constrictor of coronary arteries and there is a risk of inducing **asystole**.

12.2 Routes of administration of drugs and fluids

Umbilical venous catheterisation.
Tracheal tube (adrenaline only).
Rarely intracardiac injection.

12.2.1 Umbilical venous catheterisation

Drugs injected into a peripheral vein or directly into an umbilical cord vessel will not reach the heart quickly and may not be effective. A catheter should therefore be inserted into the umbilical vein. Blood or other colloid may also be given by this route to a baby who is shocked.

Sterile gloves should be worn and care taken with aseptic technique.

- **Place** a cotton or tape ligature loosely knotted around the base of the cord.
- **Clean** the cord quickly with chlorhexidine in water (spirit can cause skin damage), but avoid spilling disinfectant onto the skin.
- **Attach** a three-way tap and a syringe containing 5% dextrose or 0.9% sodium chloride to a FG4 or 5 umbilical catheter.
- **Fill** the catheter with fluid.

- **Cut** the umbilical cord a short distance (1–2 cm) from the skin. Grasp the edge of the cord with one of the artery forceps.
- **Identify** the three vessels. The single thin-walled vein is usually seen in the upper part of the cord and should be easy to differentiate from the two contracted white bloodless arteries which are usually found in the lower quadrants when the cord is cut relatively close to the abdominal wall (Figure 12.1).
- **Advance** the catheter into the umbilical vein. The vein may need to be dilated first with a blunt dilator but is usually easily entered using the catheter alone as a probe. Insert the catheter, handling it with the forceps, until blood can be aspirated freely. The catheter should be advanced to about 5 cm in a term baby. Beware of inserting the catheter into the liver or portal system. Injection of drugs here may cause damage. Suspect this if blood cannot be easily aspirated and withdraw the catheter until blood appears.
- **Fix** the catheter, if necessary, with a single piece of tape across the abdomen. For more permanent fixation a stitch may be used. It is usual to remove the catheter when the emergency administration of drugs or fluids is no longer required.

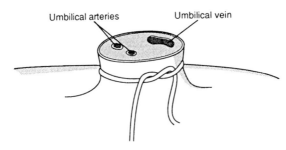

Figure 12.1. The umbilical cord prepared for venous cannulation.

12.2.2 Tracheal route

This is only suitable for administration of adrenaline and, although widely used, there is little evidence that it is effective[5]. It may be least effective if given before the lungs have been properly inflated.

- **Inject** the dose via the tracheal tube during a brief disconnection of the system.
- **Reconnect** and give four or five quick inflations before continuing ventilation in the normal way.

12.2.3 Intracardiac injection

This should not be used except in extreme circumstances. Always try umbilical venous catheterisation first.

- **Use** a 21G (green) needle on a syringe.
- **Select** a point as close as possible to the left sternal edge, between the ribs immediately below a line joining the nipples.
- **Aim** towards the spine. The needle will usually enter the right ventricle or atrium. **Check** that the needle is in a cardiac chamber by aspirating blood into the syringe. **Do not** inject unless blood can first be aspirated freely.

Alternatively, the subcostal route may be used.
- Palpate the sternocostal angle on the left.
- Insert the needle aiming at the left scapula.
- Aspirate throughout the procedure and inject after blood has been obtained.

External chest compression should recommence as soon as possible after the procedure.

13 After resuscitation

13.1 If the baby responds to resuscitation efforts

The baby may need continuing observation and thus should be admitted to the neonatal unit or transitional care unit as appropriate. This judgement will need to be made on an individual basis and advice may be needed from a more experienced member of staff. A measurement of umbilical cord blood pH and base deficit may be useful. Double clamping a section of the cord may enable a more accurate sample to be taken, usually from the umbilical vein.

13.2 If the baby fails to respond to resuscitation efforts

Where possible, the decision to abandon resuscitation efforts should be taken by an experienced member of staff, such as a specialist trainee paediatrician or a consultant. It is helpful if someone known to the parents, such as the midwife who has cared for the mother during labour, is present.

In the absence of firm evidence as to how long to persevere in the absence of a heart beat, it is suggested that resuscitation efforts should be discontinued if there has definitely not been any spontaneous cardiac output after about 20 minutes of full support. This is, however, an arbitrary time limit and individual circumstances and local practice guidelines should be taken into account.

If the baby has a spontaneous heart rate but is making no respiratory effort despite full resuscitative measures, assisted ventilation should continue until further information is available.

There are reversible causes for apnoea including iatrogenic hypocarbia or sedation due to drugs. If heart rate and peripheral pulses are good then support should be continued and the baby transferred to the neonatal unit where further assessment may be made.

Written guidelines should be available and all staff should be aware of these so that they will know how to proceed.

Resuscitation of the baby born at 24 weeks' gestation or less is considered in Section 15.7.2.

Any resuscitation procedures performed should be fully explained to the parents, together with any future plans that have been made. If resuscitation has been unsuccessful, appropriate bereavement counselling should be commenced.

14 Transfer to the neonatal unit

Local guidelines should be agreed to help decide which babies should be transferred to the neonatal unit. The criteria for admission might include gestational age, birth weight, umbilical cord blood pH or base deficit values and some, but by no means all, congenital abnormalities. If in doubt, it is always safer to transfer the baby to an area where close observation is possible.

If the neonatal unit is close by, the baby may be transferred whilst still on the resuscitation trolley provided the temperature is well maintained.

Where necessary a transport incubator should be available for this purpose. Ensure that the baby is kept warm and that the airway is secure. Monitoring facilities for heart and respiration rates and oxygen saturation should be available.

15 Special considerations

15.1 Meconium

15.1.1 Amniotic fluid lightly stained with meconium

This should not cause any problems. It is not necessary to intubate or suction well babies when the amniotic fluid has been lightly stained with meconium.

15.1.2 Amniotic fluid heavily stained with particulate meconium

This may cause two problems. Firstly, the baby may already be hypoxaemic and asphyxiated and, secondly, meconium may have been inhaled, either *in utero* or during delivery, which may cause problems with ventilation.

Aspirate the baby's mouth and nostrils gently using a wide-bore suction catheter as soon as the baby's head is delivered.

If the baby is vigorous and pink in spite of the presence of thick meconium

There is some evidence that intubating a struggling healthy baby may cause later complications and may be of no benefit[6].

Suction of the oropharynx and nostrils, if obviously containing meconium, should suffice.

*If particulate meconium is present in the liquor and the baby is **not** vigorous*

Do not suction aggressively as stimulation of the back of the pharynx may cause the baby to gasp and inhale meconium.

On the resuscitation surface, gently suck out the oropharynx and inspect the vocal cords using a laryngoscope.

If meconium is present at the cords

Intubate with as large a tracheal tube as possible.

Aspirate meconium from the trachea by applying suction directly to the tracheal tube whilst withdrawing and removing it

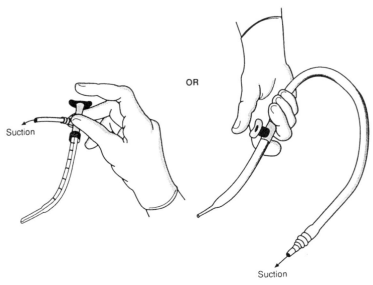

OR

Suction

Suction

Figure 15.1. Methods of tracheal suction.

(Figure 15.1). Suction through a wide-bore suction catheter passed down a large tracheal tube is a less satisfactory alternative.

Repeat these steps whilst meconium is still being aspirated.

Avoid positive pressure ventilation at this stage unless the heart rate is <60 beats per minute and decreasing.

When as much meconium as possible has been removed, **ventilate** the baby. It is useful but not vital to try to clear the airway of meconium before starting positive pressure ventilation. **Continue** normal resuscitation measures.

There is no evidence that lung lavage with normal saline confers any extra advantage and it may cause harm by removing pulmonary surfactant.

Once regular respirations are established, **remove** meconium from the stomach using a nasogastric or orogastric tube.

15.2 Pneumothorax

15.2.1 Incidence

Serious pneumothorax requiring drainage in the delivery room is very rare but may arise during resuscitation, particularly when pulmonary hypoplasia or meconium aspiration is present.

15.2.2 Clinical signs

- Asymmetry of breath sounds.
- Displacement of the cardiac impulse.
- Tense abdomen.
- Asymmetry of chest wall movement.
- Downward displacement of the liver.

If the baby is relatively well and there is doubt about the diagnosis

Transfer to the neonatal unit for further assessment.

If the baby is deteriorating

A pleural cannula should be inserted into the fourth intercostal space in the anterior axillary line. A three-way tap and syringe should be attached and the pneumothorax aspirated. An underwater seal should then be attached.

If the baby is desperately ill, insertion of a needle may decompress a pneumothorax while a chest drain is prepared, but needling the chest, particularly with a butterfly needle, on faint suspicion of a pneumothorax may itself cause a pneumothorax and be dangerous. The fact that air drains through a butterfly needle tubing does not necessarily mean that a pneumothorax was present in the first place. If available, cold light illumination in a preterm baby may help to confirm the presence of a pneumothorax.

15.3 Acute blood loss

15.3.1 Diagnosis

- Evidence of blood loss at delivery.
- Pallor and poor pulse volume.
- Poor response to resuscitation.
- Feto-maternal or feto-fetal transfusion.
- Haemolysis suspected from the history.

15.3.2 Management

- **Catheterise** the umbilical vein (see section 12.2.1).
- **Infuse** Group O Rhesus negative blood 20 ml/kg over 5–10 minutes.
- Further volume expanders should be given until the circulation is improving (Section 12.1.3).

- **Positive pressure ventilation** and external chest compression may also be required.
- **Transfer** the baby to the neonatal unit as soon as possible.
- 4·5% albumin or plasma should be given if blood is not immediately available.

15.4 Hydrops fetalis

15.4.1 Incidence

Non-immune hydrops occurs in about 1 in 3000 deliveries. Hydrops due to Rhesus D iso-immunisation is becoming very rare and the incidence is now probably about 1 in 15 000 deliveries. In the UK, most cases should be diagnosed antenatally from ultrasound scans.

These babies may be very difficult to resuscitate and experienced personnel should be present. In many cases abdominal fluid limits inflation of the lungs and requires drainage, and it is occasionally also necessary to drain the pleural cavity, particularly if hydrops is associated with a chylothorax.

15.4.2 Management

If there is tense ascites limiting inflation of the lungs

Keep the resuscitation surface tilted so that the baby is on a head-up slope.

Insert a cannula into the left iliac fossa in order to avoid puncturing the capsule of the liver or spleen.

Drain fluid slowly, removing just enough to facilitate ventilation.

If there are pleural effusions which prevent lung inflation

Insert a pleural cannula into the fourth intercostal space at the anterior axillary line.

Drain the fluid, preferably via a three-way tap and syringe.

Remember pulmonary hypoplasia may be present which will lead to difficulty in oxygenation.

Severe anaemia may be present and transfusion with Group O Rhesus negative blood 20 ml/kg, over 5–10 minutes, may be necessary. Beware volume overload – exchange transfusion may be more appropriate.

15.5 Diaphragmatic hernia

15.5.1 Incidence

1 in 3500 deliveries. 85% are left-sided.

This is often diagnosed antenatally but can still sometimes be encountered unexpectedly. The baby may be difficult to resuscitate and remain profoundly cyanosed.

15.5.2 Clinical signs

- Cyanosis.
- Scaphoid (flat) abdomen.
- Cardiac impulse on the right side of the chest.

15.5.3 Resuscitation

If possible, these babies should be delivered electively so that the appropriate resuscitation team may be forewarned and in attendance.

Do not ventilate via a mask as this will inflate the bowel and worsen the situation.

Intubate and ventilate if the baby needs resuscitation.

Empty the stomach of air using a large nasogastric tube and aspirate frequently.

If appropriate, ensure **muscle relaxation** with pancuronium (100 μg/kg), or other suitable non-depolarising muscle relaxant, to prevent the baby inflating the bowel with air.

Transfer to an appropriate neonatal unit for specialist medical and surgical care.

15.6 Severe congenital abnormality

Fetal abnormalities are now often diagnosed antenatally and a clear plan of management will have been determined in advance through discussions involving the parents, and experienced obstetric and paediatric staff. It is helpful if the paediatrician present at the delivery is someone known to the parents, who has had the opportunity to discuss the problem and the likely management beforehand. If there is a named midwife she should have been involved in these discussions and, where possible, should be present at the delivery. In all cases the midwife attending the woman during labour should be appraised of the plan of management.

Occasionally, however, a baby will be born with an unexpected severe abnormality. Unless the abnormality is really extreme, for example anencephaly, the baby should be resuscitated as decisions about further management are best made in the neonatal unit rather than hurriedly in the delivery suite. If resuscitation is difficult an experienced paediatrician should be called immediately. Remember that many abnormalities may initially seem more serious than they actually are.

15.7 The very preterm baby

15.7.1 Babies born at 25–28 weeks' gestation

The same principles of resuscitation apply to these babies as to term babies, but a preterm baby who is failing to establish regular respiration needs support given more swiftly. Periods of face mask ventilation should be brief and if these do not achieve a satisfactory response by 30–60 seconds then tracheal intubation should be carried out. A few of these small babies may need a surprisingly high inflation pressure to expand the lungs. This should be applied with careful observation of the chest wall for movement, as it is easy to induce pneumothorax or pulmonary interstitial emphysema.

Prompt respiratory support may improve the outcome and the baby must not be allowed to deteriorate during transfer to the neonatal unit.

15.7.2 Babies born at 24 weeks' gestation or less

Locally agreed **written guidelines** should be available, and should emphasise that decisions about resuscitating these babies should be made by an experienced paediatrician to whom this responsibility has been designated. The guidelines should specify when a paediatrician should attend a delivery but make it clear that active resuscitation may not be appropriate, even if the baby is born with a discernible heart beat. Where possible, the strategy should be discussed beforehand with parents and attending obstetric and midwifery staff.

Very preterm babies who are extremely bruised at delivery or who have needed adrenaline during resuscitation generally have an extremely poor outcome[7].

Very few babies of 23 weeks' gestation survive and there is a very high incidence of neurodevelopmental problems among those who do. Nevertheless, some babies of 23 weeks' gestation have survived without severe problems, so that resuscitation may be justified in those who are in good condition at birth, making sustained spontaneous respiratory efforts and are not excessively bruised. The situation must be judged individually and it is important that an experienced paediatrician is present at the delivery of any baby who is thought to be at the borderline of viability. Sometimes it is appropriate for the parents simply to hold their extremely preterm baby after delivery and it is helpful for a paediatrician to be there to explain what is happening.

If in doubt, the baby should be resuscitated and taken to the neonatal unit where decisions about further management can be made. It is usually best to judge the outlook on gestational age and condition at birth rather than birth weight, as some extremely growth retarded babies have survived normally and there is rarely time to weigh the baby in the delivery room.

16 Record keeping

16.1 Baby case notes prepared before birth

Communication can be improved if case notes with the baby's hospital number are made up before delivery, as soon as a problem has been identified. Letters can then be copied to these notes and the plan of action at delivery clearly written in them so that whenever the baby is delivered the staff are aware of what the parents expect to happen.

16.2 Details of resuscitation

The resuscitation must always be fully documented.
The record should include:

- Times to first gasp, regular respirations and heart rate.
- The mode of, and response to, resuscitation.
- Time at tracheal intubation and duration of ventilation.
- Drugs given, route and dosage.
- Umbilical cord blood pH, blood gases and base deficit.
- Names and designation of personnel present at resuscitation.
- Reasons for any delay in resuscitation.
- Information given to the parents.

The entry must be clearly timed, dated and legibly signed.

16.3 The Apgar Score

This is a description of the condition of the baby soon after birth and the response to resuscitation. It was not designed to be a predictor of neurodevelopmental outcome and should not be used as such without taking other clinical factors into account. **It is not a substitute for fully documented records.**

Clinical feature	Apgar Score		
	0	1	2
Heart rate	Nil	< 100	> 100
Respiratory effort*	Absent	Gasping or irregular	Regular or strong cry
Muscle tone	Limp	Some flexion	Active movement
Response to stimulation	Nil	Grimace	Cry or cough
Colour**	White	Blue	Pink

* If the baby is intubated the score should reflect the underlying respiratory effort of the baby and not the rate of lung inflation given by the resuscitator.
** It is common for newborn babies to have peripheral cyanosis and the central or trunk colour should be recorded.

Notes on assigning the scores

A score for each clinical feature should be assigned to the baby's status at 1, 5 and 10 minutes and at regular intervals thereafter until the baby is stable. The scores should be recorded in full and documented contemporaneously.

17 Teaching and training

It is essential that all paediatric, obstetric, midwifery and neonatal nursing staff receive training in neonatal resuscitation.

17.1 Induction programmes

New staff should have an induction programme which includes principles of resuscitation, teamwork and practice with an infant model. They should be familiar with all aspects of the equipment used on the labour wards and should know who is responsible for equipment checks. They should also be made familiar with the guidelines of the unit and the local procedure for summoning further assistance. Until new staff who will be responsible for intubating babies have successfully done so, they should be accompanied by someone who is competent in intubation.

17.2 Regular updates

Updates in resuscitation training should be available and those responsible for organising this should be clearly identified. The importance of teamwork should be emphasised and resuscitation training assignments should include exercises in working together.

17.3 Neonatal resuscitation programmes

Medical staff, midwives and neonatal nurses should be given opportunities to attend these programmes. Certificates of attendance and regular revision updates should be expected. Neonatal Advanced Life Support Courses are now available.

18 Communication with parents and other professionals

Whenever a problem has been suspected antenatally, such as congenital abnormality or threatened preterm delivery, this should be discussed before delivery with both parents by an obstetrician and a paediatrician, preferably with the named midwife present, and a plan of action decided upon. Other professionals, such as a paediatric surgeon or a geneticist may need to be involved. The general practitioner should be kept fully informed.

At delivery the plan should be adhered to and, if it is necessary to take the baby to the neonatal unit, parents should have an opportunity to touch or hold their baby first whenever possible.

If a baby needs resuscitation, parents should be kept informed of the measures that are being taken and why they are necessary. The midwife in charge of the delivery may take on this role whilst resuscitation is going on.

If a baby is unexpectedly born in a poor condition it is important to be as frank as possible without making loose or ill-informed statements about fetal distress, unwarranted assumptions or prejudgements. In particular, leave discussion about obstetric management to the senior obstetrician.

Decisions to discontinue resuscitation or to resuscitate the extremely preterm baby should also closely involve parents.

All discussions, before and after delivery, should be recorded in the case notes. Ideally, infant case notes should be available before delivery of a baby in whom a problem is anticipated.

The obstetrician and midwife responsible for the mother's care and the general practitioner should be kept informed of the baby's progress.

19 Audit

This is essential in order to assess whether guidelines are being observed and whether local practice matches accepted standards of care. Guidelines and practices should regularly be audited and reviewed.

20 Newer developments

Some units may already be using some of the techniques outlined below but they are not yet widely accepted. **It is clear that further research is needed with regard to these newer developments.**

20.1 Oxygen saturation monitoring

Although not yet widely used in delivery suites, oxygen saturation monitoring could become part of basic monitoring, particularly with the advent of the use of air/oxygen mixtures. Care must be taken with the very preterm baby where oxygen saturation measurements may fail to identify hyperoxia and put the baby at risk of reduced cerebral blood flow and retinal arterial vasospasm.

20.2 Air/oxygen mixing

There are now data suggesting that, in term babies, 100% oxygen has little advantage over air[8]. Preterm infants may have a significant reduction in cerebral blood flow if allowed to become hyperoxic[9]. If air/oxygen mixing facilities and oxygen saturation monitoring are available, it may be more appropriate to use an inspired oxygen concentration of 40% initially and then increase this if required.

20.3 Laryngeal masks

These have been used by anaesthetists with success in general resuscitation, but there is less experience in neonatal resuscitation. They may be useful when intubation is difficult in conditions such as Pierre Robin sequence but, as with all techniques, should only be used by those with specific training.

20.4 Expiratory carbon dioxide monitoring

This is currently used by anaesthetists as a standard monitoring for ventilated patients in the operating theatre.

Appendix A: Deliveries considered to be at risk

Guidelines are given here, but must be agreed locally. It should be remembered that in some situations more than one trained person will be needed and close teamwork is essential.

A.1 Situations where someone experienced in resuscitation should be present and an assistant allocated

- Significant fetal distress.
- Thick meconium staining of the amniotic fluid.
- Vaginal breech deliveries.
- Gestation that is less than 32 completed weeks.
- Serious fetal abnormality, for example diaphragmatic hernia, hydrops fetalis.
- Concern of attending staff.

A.2 Situations where someone experienced in resuscitation may be required and if not in attendance must be immediately available

It is impossible to give firm guidelines as this will depend very much on local circumstances. Potential problems should be notified to the team who will be responsible for resuscitation, even if it is not thought necessary for them to be in attendance. It is suggested that those drawing up local guidelines consider the various problems that might arise, decide the guidelines for each and ensure that those responsible for the delivery of babies are familiar with them. The sort of problems that need to be considered include rotational forceps or Ventouse delivery, multiple pregnancy, intrauterine growth retardation, evidence of maternal infection or haemorrhage, babies of 32–36 weeks' or > 42 weeks' gestation, 'softer' signs of fetal distress such as amniotic fluid lightly stained with meconium, elective caesarean section, and fetal abnormality.

Careful clinical audit will indicate the local pattern of requirements for the various levels of experience in resuscitation of the newborn.

Appendix B: Equipment

B.1 Equipment for resuscitation at home

Access to a mobile phone or telephone within the home.
A room heater and good light.
An appropriate padded surface at table height.
Towels and gloves.
Self-inflating resuscitation bag, valve and face masks of different sizes (Sections B.5.2, B.5.3, B.5.4).
Suction device and catheters.
Resuscitation flow chart.
Stop watch.
Stethoscope.
Oxygen cylinder with regulated flow rate of up to 10 L/min and an adjustable pressure-relief valve within the system.
Syringes, needles and disposal box.
Checklist.

B.2 Equipment for resuscitation in hospital

This is a suggested list of what should be available in each delivery room and in the accident and emergency department:
A resuscitation surface.
An overhead radiant heat source.
Towels and gloves.
Stop clock.
Stethoscope.
Suction device and catheters.
Oxygen/air supply with variable regulated flow rate and adjustable pressure-relief valve (Section B.5.1).
Y-piece or 500-ml self-inflating resuscitation bag, valve and face masks (Sections B.5.2, B.5.3, B.5.4).
Two laryngoscopes with straight, appropriate size blades, spare bulbs and batteries (Section B.5.5).
Tracheal tubes (2·5, 3·0, 3·5 and 4·0 mm), introducers and connectors (Section B.5.6).

Magill forceps if using nasal route for intubation.
Syringes, needles and disposal box.
Scissors.
Adhesive tape.
Umbilical vessel catheterisation pack (Section B.5.7).
Nasogastric tube sizes 5 and 8.
Oropharyngeal airways, sizes 00 and 0.
Intravenous cannulae.
Pleural cannula set.
Checklist.
Resuscitation Charts 1 and 2 (pp 57–58).

B.3 Drugs and fluids

Adrenaline – 1:10 000 (100 μg/ml).
Dextrose – 5% and 10% (10 ml ampoules).
Sodium bicarbonate – 4·2% (or 8·4% diluted with an equal volume of 5–10% dextrose).
Sodium chloride – 0·9%.
Access to a volume expander (plasma; albumin; Group O Rhesus negative blood).
Naloxone – 400 μg/ml.
Water for injection – for adrenaline dilution.

B.4 Post resuscitation equipment needs after high-risk deliveries

Transport incubator.
ECG/respiration monitor.
Temperature monitor.
Oxygen saturation monitor.
Transcutaneous oxygen monitor.
Easy access to neonatal intensive care or special care baby unit.

B.5 Further notes on equipment

B.5.1 In resuscitation it has been traditional to use an inspired oxygen concentration of 100%, although there are now data challenging this (Section 20.2).

B.5.2 Face masks

Masks must be circular with a soft deformable edge. They should preferably be made of a clear material such as silicone. Three sizes should be available, and where small premature babies are to be delivered, a small size mask will be needed. It is essential that a seal is achieved between the mask and the face in order to achieve satisfactory ventilation during resuscitation.

B.5.3 Y-piece system

With a Y-piece system, a finger is used to occlude the exhalation port and oxygen is delivered to the face mask from a pressurised oxygen supply via an adjustable pressure-limiting safety valve preset to 30–40 cmH$_2$O. The circuit should include a manometer.

B.5.4 Self-inflating resuscitation bag

An alternative to the Y-piece system is a self-inflating resuscitation bag.

The standard neonatal self-inflating resuscitation bag has a volume of about 250 ml. The ventilation volume can be increased by using a bag with a 500 ml capacity which allows inflation pressure to be maintained for > 1 second. Poor performance of resuscitation bag and mask ventilation may be related to the short inspiratory time provided by the smaller device[10]. Beware of delivering excessive volumes when the larger volume bag is attached to a tracheal tube.

B.5.5 Laryngoscopes

A straight blade design is preferable and the blade size should be appropriate for the size of the baby. There are many designs available and it is best to become practised with one design. A second laryngoscope, spare bulbs and batteries should be available.

B.5.6 Tracheal tubes (Figure B.1)

Tracheal tubes may be either straight sided or shouldered. Most tubes have a black vocal cord depth of intubation guideline near the tip. The straight sided tubes may be used with an introducer or stylet. If an introducer is used it should be shaped to conform with the curve of the tube and should not protrude beyond the tip.

The size of tracheal tube should be selected according to the anticipated weight or gestation of the baby:

- Size 3·0–3·5 for > 2000 g or > 34 weeks.

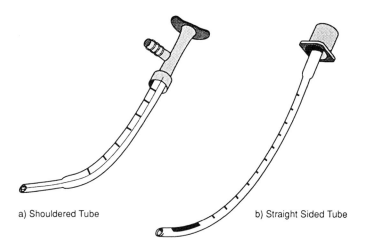

a) Shouldered Tube   b) Straight Sided Tube

Figure B.1. Tracheal tubes.

- Size 2·5–3·0 for 750–2000 g or 26–34 weeks.
- Size 2·5* for < 750 g or < 26 weeks.

OR as a guideline:

- Tracheal tube size (mm) = Gestational age/10.

Note: all sizes relate to internal diameter (mm).

When a large baby requires intubation, particularly one who has inhaled meconium, use the largest possible size of tube which safely achieves intubation without undue force.

---

* A size 2·0 tracheal tube should **not** be used as it is very difficult to achieve effective ventilation because of the internal resistance.

B.5.7 Umbilical vessel catheterisation pack

The basic pack should contain a linen ligature, scalpel blade, graduated 4FG end-hole umbilical catheter with a luer lock, three-way tap, 2-ml syringe, two artery forceps, one fine artery dilator, sterile towel, gauze squares and suture pack.

Appendix C: Equipment checks

All equipment, gases, drugs and fluids should be checked by a designated member of the delivery suite staff at the start of each midwifery shift and after each resuscitation procedure. The responsibility for this should be agreed locally. Any reusable equipment should be cleaned and sterilised. The individual attending a delivery who is responsible for the resuscitation of the baby should check that all the equipment is present and functioning. The checks required are detailed below:

1. Any overhead or other **heating** device is functioning and the temperature within the delivery room is at least 25°C.
2. Warm dry **towels**, a **hat** for the baby and **sterile gloves** for the staff are available in the delivery room.
3. The **clock** is functioning.
4. The **suction** device is functioning with a negative pressure of 100 mmHg (13.3 kPa).
5. There is an **oxygen supply** capable of providing flow rates up to 10 L/min. All oxygen cylinders contain sufficient oxygen for a resuscitation procedure.
6. Any **pressure-limiting device** for face mask or tracheal resuscitation is working and set at a prescribed maximum level, usually 30 cmH$_2$O.
7. Resuscitation equipment is available, including **Y-piece** or appropriate-sized **bag, masks** and, in hospitals, a range of **tracheal tubes** and **introducers** (if used). The agreed range of **drugs** and **fluids** must be available, their expiry dates checked, together with a supply of **syringes** and **needles** and **cannulae**. Check in particular that the **laryngoscope** functions and a **second laryngoscope, spare bulbs** and **batteries** are available.
8. All **ventilation devices** are connectable to face masks and tracheal tubes.

References

1. British Paediatric Association. *Neonatal Resuscitation* London: The British Paediatric Association 1993.
2. Royal College of Obstetricians and Gynaecologists. *Working Party Report on HIV Infection in Maternity Care and Gynaecology.* London: Royal College of Obstetricians and Gynaecologists, 1990.
3. David R. Closed chest cardiac massage in the newborn infant. *Pediatrics* 1988; **81**: 552–554.
4. Todres ID, Rogers MC. Methods of external cardiac massage in the newborn infant. *Pediatrics* 1975; **86**: 781–782.
5. Lindemann R. Resuscitation of the newborn. Endotracheal administration of epinephrine. *Acta Paediatr Scand* 1984; **73**: 210–212.
6. Linder N, Aranda JV, Tsur M et al. Need for endotracheal intubation in meconium-stained neonates. *J Pediatr* 1988; **112**: 613–615.
7. Sims DG, Heal CA, Bartle SM. Use of adrenaline and atropine in neonatal resuscitation. *Arch Dis Child* 1994; **70**: F3–F10.
8. Ramji S, Ahuja S, Thiupuram S et al. Resuscitation of asphyxic newborn infants with room air or 100% oxygen. *Pediatr Res* 1993; **34**: 809–812.
9. Lundstrom KE, Pryds O, Greisen G. Oxygen at birth and prolonged cerebral vasoconstriction in preterm infants. *Arch Dis Child* 1995; **73**: F81–F86.
10. Milner AD. Resuscitation of the newborn. *Arch Dis Child* 1991; **66**: 66–69.

Recommended reading

Chameides L, Hazinski M, eds. *Pediatric Advanced Life Support*. Dallas: American Heart Association, 1994.

Dawes GS. *Foetal and Neonatal Physiology*. Chicago: Year Book Medical Publishers, 1968.

European Resuscitation Council. *Recommendations for Resuscitation of the Newly Born*, April 1997.

Halliday HL. Meconium aspiration syndrome. In: Sinclair JC, Bracken MB, eds. *Effective Care of the Newborn Infant*. Oxford: Oxford University Press, 1991; pp 370–373.

Peliowski A, Finer N. Resuscitation of the term infant at birth. In: Sinclair JC, Bracken MB, eds. *Effective Care of the Newborn Infant*. Oxford: Oxford University Press, 1991; pp 253–255.

Richmond S, ed. Northern Neonatal Network. *Principles of Resuscitation at Birth*. Newcastle upon Tyne: Hindson Print, 1996.

Tyson J, Silverman W, Reisch J. Immediate care of the newborn infant. In: Chalmers I, Enkin M, Keirse M, eds. *Effective Care in Pregnancy and Childbirth*. Oxford: Oxford University Press, 1991; pp 1293–1312.

Walker AM. Circulatory transitions at birth and the control of the neonatal circulation. In: Hanson MA, Spencer J, Rodeck C, eds. *Fetus and Neonate*, Vol 1. Cambridge: Cambridge Univcersity Press, 1993; pp 160–196.

Resuscitation Chart 1

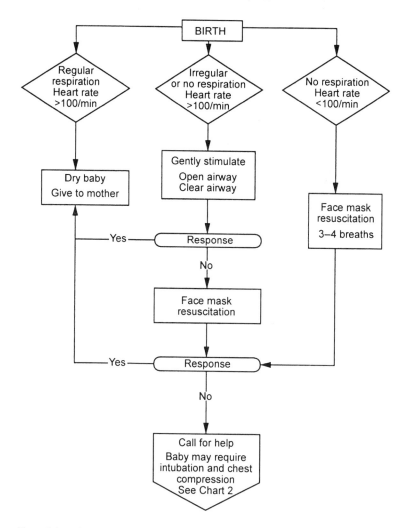

Note: If there is particulate meconium and the baby is unresponsive, proceed at once to Chart 2.

Resuscitation Chart 2

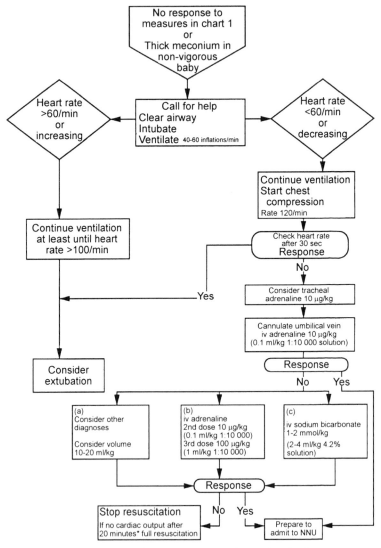

No response to measures in chart 1
or
Thick meconium in non-vigorous baby

Heart rate >60/min or increasing

Call for help
Clear airway
Intubate
Ventilate 40-60 inflations/min

Heart rate <60/min or decreasing

Continue ventilation
Start chest compression
Rate 120/min

Continue ventilation at least until heart rate >100/min

Check heart rate after 30 sec
Response

No

Consider tracheal adrenaline 10 µg/kg

Yes

Cannulate umbilical vein
iv adrenaline 10 µg/kg
(0.1 ml/kg 1:10 000 solution)

Response

No   Yes

Consider extubation

(a)
Consider other diagnoses

Consider volume 10-20 ml/kg

(b)
iv adrenaline
2nd dose 10 µg/kg
(0.1 ml/kg 1:10 000)
3rd dose 100 µg/kg
(1 ml/kg 1:10 000)

(c)
iv sodium bicarbonate
1-2 mmol/kg
(2-4 ml/kg 4.2% solution)

Response

No   Yes

Stop resuscitation
If no cardiac output after 20 minutes* full resuscitation

Prepare to admit to NNU

(a) Consider whilst preparing for (b) +/- (c) depending on local policy.
*May vary with individual circumstances and local guidelines.
IV = intravenous; NNU = neonatal unit.

Index